The Heart of the Matter

The Heart of the Matter

A New Beginning

Felicia Pharagood-Wade, MD

iUniverse, Inc.
New York Lincoln Shanghai

The Heart of the Matter
A New Beginning

iUniverse books may be ordered through booksellers or by contacting:

iUniverse
2021 Pine Lake Road, Suite 100
Lincoln, NE 68512
www.iuniverse.com
1-800-Authors (1-800-288-4677)

ISBN-13: 978-0-595-39327-5 (pbk)
ISBN-13: 978-0-595-83723-6 (ebk)
ISBN-10: 0-595-39327-6 (pbk)
ISBN-10: 0-595-83723-9 (ebk)

Printed in the United States of America

First Giving Honor to God who is the Head and the Love of my Life

I thank you for all your blessings to me. I appreciate every thing you have done for me.

You have taught me such wondrous things and specifically that you are the Smart one and the Great Physician

I dedicate this book to the second love love of my life, my husband, David Wade

Thank you for teaching me about unconditional love, fallacies, acceptance, sacrifice, generosity, leadership, forgiveness and that love should not hurt.

To my daughter, Amanda, you are the heart of the matter, Thank you for teaching me about love, the unselfish love of Christ, self sacrificing love, where all you want is the good for the other person. The legacy that I leave you is to love God with all your heart, do not be a know it all, find a good husband and love him with all your heart, tithe, it is not your money you owe it to God, save something for a rainy day, spend something on yourself sometimes, not all the time, and lend a helping hand.

To my mother, There are no words to say thank you for all that you have done. I can never say thank you enough times for all the love that you have shown me my entire life to where I grew up feeling loved, smart, and wealthy when I know that you went without many times trying to take care of us as a young widow.

To my sister, my best friend

To my nephew, te yamo embrace who you are and thank God for it.

To my uncle, thank you for being there in Daddy's absence

To my family, The Pharagoods, the Alstons, the Wades and Latimers(Barbara☺) I love you all.

Contents

Acknowledgements

I have to acknowledge my Pastor and first Lady as an impetus to move forward. You received my daughter and I with such open arms that words are difficult to find to articulate my gratitude. It is a pleasure to tithe to the ministry at VOF because the Pastor does not brag about how many jets he owns, or how many carats his wife is wearing, he brags about how much he loves his members and then shows it by caring for them through 55 ministries as well as Hurricane Katrina members.

I have to acknowledge Ebenezer Baptist Church, The church with a loving heart. Thank you for all the love and teaching me stewardship. Pastor Roberts, it is well.

Introduction

One out of every 4 people are overweight or obese. The definition of overweight is more than 20 pounds over your recommended weight based upon your height and body habitus. This statistic has increased in the past 20 years due to the availability of low cost high fat, high salt and high sugar foods.

Body mass index (BMI), expressed as weight/height^2 (BMI; kg/m^2), is commonly used to classify overweight (BMI 25.0-29.9) and obesity (BMI greater than or equal to 30.0) among adults (age 20 years and over).

As a result of the obesity epidemic in this country, the morbidity and mortality for the average American have increased. Adipose tissue according to recent studies increases the risk of, cardiovascular, breast cancer, and other diseases.

Abdominal obesity, cortisol, sleep deprivation and stress are interrelated and the research is evolving.

Over a billion dollars in lost productivity occurs every year due to the illnesses caused by obesity. The economic impact from co-morbid conditions such as hypertension, diabetes, cardiovascular disease is staggering.

Obesity affects every organ system in the body including the brain—example depression. It accounts for cardiovascular problems even when you have 0 trans fat in your food. Heart disease is the leading cause of death, killing over 500,000 Americans per year. It costs this country over 500 billion dollars a year in lost wages and employee productivity due to the increased disability due to joint and back problems, adult onset diabetes, hypertension, headaches and gallbladder disease. This issue is beyond the scope of this book, however it is one that will continually need to be addressed from a public health perspective.

Overindulgent, erratic, and emotional eating in response to pain, anger, frustration, happiness or boredom typically represent some of the environmental factors that contribute to obesity in addition to genetic predisposition, and organic disorders. The discipline and willingness to change one's eating, exercise, and life style habits are the most significant factors in predicting success. Behavior modification is the key. Not just making the food behave. It is essential to make a conscious decision to eat to live and not to live to eat. We must begin to understand when we are eating in response to another trigger and when we really are hungry.

Chapter 1

The Obesity Epidemic

- 58 Million Overweight; 40 Million Obese; 3 Million morbidly Obese
- Eight out of 10 over 25's Overweight
- 78% of American's not meeting basic activity level recommendations
- 25% completely Sedentary
- 76% increase in Type II diabetes in adults 30–40 yrs old since 1990

Obesity Related Diseases

- 80% of type II diabetes related to obesity
- 70% of Cardiovascular disease related to obesity
- 42% breast and colon cancer diagnosed among obese individuals

- 30% of gall bladder surgery related to obesity
- 26% of obese people having high blood pressure

Childhood Obesity Running Out of Control

- 4% overweight 1982 | 16% overweight 1994
- 25% of all white children overweight 2001
- 33% African American and Hispanic children overweight 2001
- Hospital costs associated with childhood obesity rising from $35 Million (1979) to $127 Million (1999)

Childhood Metabolic and Heart Risks

- New study suggests one in four overweight children is already showing early signs of type II diabetes (impaired glucose intolerance)
- 60% already have one risk factor for heart disease

Surge in Childhood Diabetes

- Between 8%–45% of newly diagnosed cases of childhood diabetes are type II, associated with obesity.

- Whereas 4% of Childhood diabetes was type II in 1990, that number has risen to approximately 20%

- Depending on the age group (Type II most frequent 10–19 group) and the racial/ethnic mix of group stated

- Of Children diagnosed with Type II diabetes, 85% are obese

The definition of obesity is a disease of excess body fat characterised by a body mass index of 30+. In adults, the Body Mass Index (BMI) is the standard diagnostic tool for measuring mild obesity (BMI 30+), morbid obesity (BMI 40+), and malignant obesity (BMI 50+).-.

The risk factors and contributory causes of obesity—include a range of well-documented genetic and environmental factors. The relative effect of these causes on the development of obesity, remains unclear as the research is still evolving.

Six million American adults are now morbidly obese (BMI 40+), almost twice as high as 1980 severe obesity rates, while another 9.6 million have a BMI of 35-40. The percentage of overweight children 6–11 has nearly doubled since the early 1980's. (Source: US Census 2000; NHANES III data estimates). Additionally, the fact that each succeeding generation is heavier than the last indicates that changes in our environment are playing the key role.

Obesity tends to run in families, suggesting a genetic link. Yet families also share common dietary, physical exercise, attitude and lifestyle habits that may also contribute to obesity. Separating these from purely genetic factors is not an easy statistical or diagnostic task. Genes affect a number of weight-related processes in the body, such as metabolic rate, blood glucose metabolism, fat-storage, hormones, to name but a few. Also, some studies of adopted children indicate that adopted children tend to develop weight problems similar to their biological, rather than adoptive, parents. In addition, infants born to overweight mothers have been found to be less active and to gain more weight by the age of three months when compared with infants of normal weight mothers, suggesting a possible inborn drive to conserve energy. Research has also shown that normal-weight children of obese parents may have a lower metabolic rate than normal-weight children of non-obese parents, which can lead to weight problems in adulthood. All of this suggests that a predisposition to obesity can be inherited.

Overconsumption, eating too many calories for our basal energy requirements is another contributing factor toward the obesity epidemic. According to Dr. Marion Nestle, Professor and Chair of the Department of Nutrition and Food Studies at New York University, US agribusiness now produces 3,800 calories of food a day for every American, 500 calories more than 30 years ago—but at much lower per-calorie costs. Increases in consumption of calorie-dense foods, as evidenced by the growth of fast-food chains and higher soft drink consumption, also point to a higher energy-intake.

The type of food eaten may be a factor in the rise of obesity. Researchers continue to discover more metabolic and digestive disorders resulting from overconsumption of trans-fats and refined white flour carbohydrates, combined with low fiber intake. These eating patterns are known to interfere with food and energy metabolism in the body, and cause excessive fat storage. Associated health disorders include insulin resistance, type 2 diabetes as well as obesity.

The incidence of these "modern" diseases is increasing worldwide.

People who eat more calories need to burn more calories, otherwise their calorie surplus is stored as fat. For example, if we eat 100 more food calories a day than we burn, we gain about 1 pound in a month. That's about 10 pounds in a year.

Chapter 2

The Heart of the Matter

Overweight and obese individuals are at increased risk for many diseases and health conditions, including the following:

- Hypertension
- Dyslipidemia (for example, high total cholesterol or high levels of triglycerides)
- Type 2 diabetes
- Coronary heart disease
- Stroke
- Gallbladder disease
- Osteoarthritis
- Sleep apnea and respiratory problems
- Some cancers (endometrial, breast, and colon)

The first step in problem resolution is to discuss the matter. The heart of the matter is that it really is a matter of the heart. Writing this book made me take a look at everything that medicine does, our patient encounters, what we discuss, what we don't discuss, the patient's perception of the quality or lack of quality in the encounter, needs met and unmet, what and how we advise our patients.Often we are not the example of health that our patients look for. I can recall a teacher telling me that she was told by her gynecologist to decrease the use of estrogens due to the possible linkage between cardiovascular disease and stroke. Then she shared that she was looking for a new physician because her doctor died of a stroke. It is important to demonstrate the behavior, as well as discuss it because over 90% of our communication is nonverbal. It is no longer an era of do as I say, we are in the era of do I do. We have to thrive and the way to thrive is with God leading the way because he has given us access to all of the knowledge required to live a healthy lifestyle. It simply becomes a choice based upon a mindset and change of heart. People often make their health decisions based upon numerous factors unrelated to the direct treatment of an illness. For instance, it has to be discussed with patients what medications will cause them to gain weight if they are diabetic or have lupus requiring long term steroid use. It has to be discussed with patients what environmental factors are impacting their illness and making it difficult to get to the health and prosperity that God designed and wished for us to have above all else.

The heart of the matter is that, it is a matter of the heart in so many ways. What is the connection between cardiovascular disease, obesity, and stress? Heart disease is the leading cause of death, killing over 500,000 Americans per year. The heart of the matter is that someone's father, mother, grandmother, son, daughter has to die unnecessarily even with the availability of all the latest medical technological advances and research because of an inability to control the environmental factors of stress, eating, and a fast-paced lifestyle. Some people will have an untimely death due to hereditary cardiovascular disorders and familial hypercholesterolemia if not well controlled with medication. That is, however, not the situation in the majority of cases. Most people really refuse to believe that God made them special and that they need to take care of themselves sometimes before they can take care of someone else. That may mean getting 15 minutes rest on a plane when someone else would rather talk, not eating the angus beef for the 4th time this week, or actually getting their blood pressure checked at a fire station. It may mean taking a break even when your to do list says you can't because you have so many items to complete. It may mean taking some Tylenol for a headache instead of saying you don't like medication, instead of becoming angry that the five year old on the plane won't be completely quiet thus placing undue stress on your heart through the elevation of your blood pressure. The heart of the matter is that there are practical activities that don't take a lot of time or cost a lot of money to improve your health.

For some of us it is the disease of affluence and for others it is the disease of entitlement, I did not have it when I was younger, I am going to have it now. Sometimes, it just easier to eat 7 cookies rather than put on the running shoes, just easier to buy a bigger size and say that he or she should love me no matter what. The heart of the matter is that we really should love him or her enough to take good care of ourselves. No one should have to worry about their loved one having a heart attack in the middle of the night due to a lack of self-control or an unwillingness to monitor their health or stop smoking knowing their family history. What is the legacy of health that we are leaving for our families and children? The heart of the matter is that we owe it to God to take care of the temple that He gave us and not just put anything into it or just do anything with it, such as not getting enough rest, drinking, smoking.

Writing this book made me take a look at everything that medicine does, we just tell patients what to do, we don't show them and the way to show them is by doing not by saying. It is no longer do as I say, we are in the era of do I do. We have to thrive and the way to thrive is with God. People are making their health decisions based upon factors unrelated to the direct treatment of an illness. For instance, it has to be discussed with patient what medications will cause them to gain weight. It has to be discussed with patient what environmental factors are impacting their illness and making it difficult to get to the health and prosperity that God designed and wished above all else for us to have and take part in.

Chapter 3

Stress Don't Do a Slow Boil
What are you eating/What's Eating
At you?

It is not just about what you weigh, it is about what is weighing you down. People eat or do not eat for so many reasons. For some eating is related to stress, boredom, or pleasure.

Once you decide to address the why you eat, it becomes easier to balance the what, how, and when you eat. Unless there is an organic etiology such as diabetes, a thyroid disorder, or metabolic disorder, the weight will begin to change.

Prolonged and sustained stress often leads to distress. Unmanaged distress often impacts our somatic systems often leading to disease as a result of the dis-ease.

So many of us have unresolved matters and issues from our childhood and young adulthood which impact our lifestyle, ability and manner of handling stress, including our eating pattern. How many of us have to finish all the food on our plates because we were told that people are starving in other countries? How many of use food as comfort for the lack of attention or love?

Whatever the issue or thought, it broadcasts subliminal messages into our conscious and subconciousness, perpetuating the feelings of loneliness, anger, and sadness which fuel our desire to eat or not eat, numb ourselves with food or another addiction. I am not hypothesizing that is the only reason we eat.

Look at your food diary when you are stressed. If you like junk food when you are stressed, you tend to eat simple carbohydrates to feel better and seemingly give you energy until you crash from decreasing blood sugar levels. When stressed we don't just eat one slice of cake, we often continue in a mindless, emotionally numb-ing fashion eating to take the pain away, much like drinking, gambling, shopping, exercising, or any other addiction which offers momentary temporary satisfaction.

It is important to remember that daily life has its share of frustrations from traffic to waiting in line to getting to the airport and having to have the same credit card to confirm your ticket when you have the reservation number in hand, yet the kiosk says seek assistance.

Frustrations from the automated 411 service which never seems to be able to get you the correct number on the first call without switching over to a live operator who tells you that the number cannot be located, only to have you call back and find the number after you have paid for the 411 call twice. It's frustrating to sit in traffic get to the gas station and the gas station is out of gas, have your employer tell you that they are doing a direct deposit and they do a paper check. However if we eat because of what's eating at us we will very quickly be unable to fit into our size 6, 12, 18 jeans for women or size 34, 38, 42 waist pants jeans for men. We will also find ourselves having to deal with the co-morbidities of obesity, gallstones, arthritis, diabetes, heart disease, hypertension, back pain from truncal or abdominal obesity, sleeping difficulties, sleep apnea, and depression because obesity has an effects on many of our organ systems.

Part of decreasing your stress is to realize that you cannot carry it all on your shoulders. You cannot carry it all on your back either. Does it all have to be done now, at this moment? Can you really stomach it or does the stress show up somewhere else? You cannot carry it all, even if you make it look easy because, it shows up somewhere, high blood pressure, headaches, weight gain, weight loss, fatigue.

Many of us stress over what we cannot change, or we stress waiting for change, we do not place it in God's hands or on His time clock.

Chapter 4

Diet Schmiet—Lose weight without dieting; Eat to live not live to eat

Aren't you sick of dieting to lose weight every January after eating all through the holidays or April in time for summer, just to regain it? Sick and tired of gaining and relosing the same 10–25 pounds every year just to fit into those special jeans or an outfit to go to a special event only to regain it when life takes twists and turns or returns to normal. Aren't you sick and tired of being sick and tired?

Are you dying to be thin, taking diet pills because you are not willing to accept God's help and discipline so you want the quick way no matter that you can damage your heart and other organ systems irreversibly?

Are you eating to live or do you live to eat?

Have you already thought about what you are going to eat for dinner or tomorrow's lunch before the day is through. Is this beyond being organized, doing the grocery shopping? Is your happiest thought related to food, how it looks, smells, and tastes? Has food become your other god, your idol, the one you turn to when you are sad, depressed, tired, happy, bored, lonely, or in need of a libido adjustment.

If you are constantly bowing down to the idol god of food in gluttony and not eating in moderation or balance, you will experience a change in your health status that you did not anticipate. Don't believe me, ask people who were thin when they were young, could eat what ever they wanted, never put limits on their food nor exercised and now they have to worry about their mid section expanding and can't figure out why? Could it possibly be that it is not so much what you eat as how much? The heart of the matter is that you must burn off more than you put in your system or it will be deposited as adipose tissue due to the excess caloric intake in the majority of people. There will always be an exception, someone who has the ability to eat whatever they want and not seem to gain a pound. However, I want to assert that it is the overall health of the temple that is relevant, not just the size 2 dress. People with BMI's below 25 can still develop cardiovascular disease and strokes if they are not aware of the implications that some foods have on our blood pressure and cholesterol.

Eating in moderation determines balance. It is not about just losing weight. It is about customizing your eating and movement plan to your body habitus (whether endomorph or ectomorph),* temperament and lifestyle. The result of moderation and customization is lifelong weight management. Study naturally thin people, they have a specific regimen even though it seems like they

---

* The **endomorphic** body type is centered around the <u>digestive system</u> and is easily <u>overweight</u>. The endomorphic person also has a *visceral* temperament, which means that they are tolerant, love comfort and luxury, and are <u>extroverted</u>-in short he or she loves food and people. The jolly person

The **mesomorphic** body type is centered around muscle and the <u>circulatory system</u> and has well developed muscles. The mesomorphic person has a *somatotonic* temperament, and is courageous, energetic, active, dynamic, assertive, aggressive, competitive, and often a risk taker. The athletic person.

The **ectomorphic** body type is centered around the <u>brain</u> and nerves. These people are slim and possibly <u>underweight</u>. The ectomorphic person has a *cerebrotonic* temperament, and is artistic, sensitive, apprehensive and highly self-aware. The person may be introverted at times.

don't. Some of them have one large meal a day and they run, others eat several huge meals, however they never sit down, they are always doing something so their metabolism kicks in, other eat smaller meals or only eat when they are hungry, if they overeat, they eat in moderation the next time, they know how to cut back. Still, others get a workout in no matter what and as a result, they can eat whatever they want without gaining unwanted extra pounds. The motto is diet schmiet because diets don't work to develop lifelong habits as the majority of people can only follow a diet for a prescribed period of time and then they return to the pattern that is ingrained. Most people cannot eat a low carbohydrate diet the rest of their life. I am not saying that they are not effective initially, I am stating that at some point stress or a hormonal change will occur prompting a craving for a stress relieving food with salt or sugar. The individual on the low carbohydrate diet may find that giving in to such a craving will cause them to plateau or regain some of the weight previously lost. As more and research occurs in the field of obesity it will become evident that many diet shakes, pills, and bars are not the panacea that they purport to be.Many of the ingredients have not been approved by the FDA. I am not saying don't buy them, I advocate being an informed consumer by reading and asking questions. Ask yourself, will I be able to eat this chocolate tasting bar every day for lunch the rest of my life while I watch my friends have soup and salad, spaghetti, or chicken and broccoli?

Whether you are trying to lose weight or maintain your weight, you must improve your eating habits. Eat a variety of foods, especially pasta, rice, whole meal bread, and other whole-grain foods. Balance your fat-intake. You should also eat lots of fruits and vegetables.

Remember, God made all shapes and sizes. Be good to the temple that He gave you. It is not about being a size 2 or 22. The real question is are you being good to your temple? After you have been examined by your physician and not found to have an organic disorder such as hypothyroidism for the etiology of the weight gain or inability to lose weight, ask yourself this question…Does God really want you to be a size 2 or 22 at the cost of your health? Have you decided that this is the one area of your life that you will not seek His guidance in?

If you know you have high blood pressure, monitor it, pray about how you handle stress and your lifestyle and don't have the saltiest food that you can possibly eat everyday. Do you have to have the fried chicken, fried fish or pigs feet everyday? Your body is a barometer of your commitment to health. We make commitments to everything and everyone else, why not make a commitment to the health of the temple that God gave you, so that you can achieve His greatest desire for you? He said in His Word, Beloved, I wish above all else that you may prosper and be in good health. That means have you had your dental check up this year? Have you had your mammogram, pap smear, or prostate checked? Are you watching the salt intake? Are you resting, taking your vitamins, not overloading your schedule, not trying to control everything and everybody?

Chapter 5

Mind, Body, and Spirit: An integration

For your body to exhibit it, your mind and spirit have to be balanced. It is a step by step daily process. The first step is acknowledging that God has a process and an order for every stage of life. Ask Him to enlighten you about your body…not the spot areas that you wish were different, the areas of preventive health and wellness where you have not met the goal. Is it in the area of oral health, failing to brush and floss regularly, stopping caffeine and smoking which stain the teeth in the first place, bi annual exams of the teeth with a good dentist who can empower and educate. Is it in the area of podiatric health, taking care of your feet(vaseline and socks, clipping your nails, for diabetics, annual podiatry exams and good shoes, not having people work on your feet who don't practice the state approved and specified hygenic practice. Is it dermatological health, the hands, elbow, knees, and the face, using the appropriate anti acne products as well as decreasing the internalization of stress, wearing too much camouflage makeup everyday even though it says hypoallergenic noncomdogenic, wear a little concealer or light powder and go.

Save the overall makeup for specific events. Remember to wash your face twice a day morning and evening to get the makeup off, drink plenty of water as long as you don't have an organic disorder such as kidney disease. Are you checking your breast in the shower and getting annual mammograms on your birthday? When was your last prostate, pap or pelvic exam. Are you truly practicing safe sex, not having unprotected sex no matter how wonderful the outside person looks.

The Mind

Distress and distraction can be synergistic. Meaning that when the world becomes to heavy we eat to distract us from all we have to do, need to do, want to do or must do.

Is your mind too cluttered with to do lists?

Do you have so many things to do that you are constantly distracted from what really needs to be done and feel as if you are going in circles and never really get anything completely done to your satisfaction? Wait on God's timing…He will show you when it is the most opportune time to get it done and how to get it done efficiently. Write it down, pray about, leave it to Him and watch your to do list dwindle.

The Body

No more excuses. Get permission from your doctor to engage in physicial activity and then walk up the stairs, walk outside, run, engage in some form of exercise every day or every other day for 30 minutes. Each day move a little more everyday than you did yesterday and rest on your Sabbath, Saturday or Sunday. Strength training is essential to stem the tide of osteoporosis, the thinning of the bones dues to muscle loss. Bones weaken as they are asked to carry less and less weight.

Dr. Huber of Tufts University has shown the benefits of weight training in her research. Losing as little as 7–10 percent of your body weight if your BMI is over 26 may improve many of the problems linked to being overweight, such as high blood pressure and diabetes.

The Spirit

Nurture your spirit, not through some selfish ritual, through prayer, meditating on the Word of God and releasing to Him everything that would weigh your spirit down and ultimately the body. The heart of the matter is to refuse to let others weigh down your spirit through their words or actions Know ye not that your Body is the Temple of the Holy Spirit.

Chapter 6

So...What's the Solution Practical Solutions—Managing your personal health risk factors, wellness planning Getting through the holidays

The method of intervention depends on your level of obesity, overall health condition, and motivation to lose weight.

Slow and steady weight loss of no more than 1–2 pounds per week is the safest way to lose weight. Too rapid weight loss can cause you to lose muscle rather than fat. It also increases your chances of developing other problems, such as gallstones and nutrient deficiencies. Losing weight rapidly is no guarantee that weight loss is likely to be permanent. Making long-term changes in your eating and physical activity habits is the only way to lose weight and keep it off!

The 10 steps

Just Follow the steps one day at a time…each day ask God to help you integrate your mind, body, and spirit through incorporating these steps in your everyday routine.

1. Reverence, Reflect, Read, Request, Replenish

    Psalms 139:23-24 Prayer for guidance and direction. We don't know everything Life is full of complexities, quagmires, and snake pits. We need a Project Manager who knows more than we do. Look at what God has created, salmon cream cheese, spinach wih peaches and raspberry yogurt dressing, rocky road or banana cream pie ice cream, peanut butter and jelly, 52 story buildings, the body with its intricate biochemical processes designed to function synergistically. Obviously, He knows more than we do.

2. Replenish your soul with His Word and with H20—Study to show thyself approved. Learn all you can and then apply it. Water will also decrease your appetite. Approximately

64–70 ounces a day unless you have water intolerance, chf, renal disease, diabetes insipidus

3. Replace nutritional deficiencies—your body is designed to crave what it needs

4. Run walk/get moving—Try to do at least 30 minutes of physical activity a day on most days of the week. The activity does not have to be done all at once. It can be done in stages: 10 minutes here, 20 minutes there, providing it adds up to 30 minutes a day.

5. Rest so that you can

6. Relax so that you can

7. Release so that you can

8. Relate—love your neighbor as yourself

9. Respond to the needs of your body your temple-in other words don't starve yourself, eat, just don't be a glutton—The food will be there, satisfy your palate and taste and move on to complete more important activities, really taste your food. Don't just eat the macaroni and cheese because it is macaroni and cheese, eat if because it tastes good. No refined sugar doing the workweek

Temperance in all things No eating 2–3 hours before bed, organize something you have been putting off for 15 minutes, relax close your eyes, write in your journal, do something for yourself, your neighbor, your husband or your child in reverse order☺

10. Relinguish control/Remember God Orders your steps

There is healing power in Jesus. He is the great physician and the Balm in Gilead.

He has all the answers like Mark Rubin said, he gave you the Maker's diet. You see I am not touting one book over the other. Choose the one that meet the requirements that you believe God has for you.As a consumer advocate of weight management programs, I would like to point out basic tenets that should be followed when selecting a program and admonish that the program should be lifelong and centered on basic health principles that can be followed consistently over a long period of time, not just for 30 days and then the weight is regained at a higher rate and the discouragement has mounted significantly. Bottom line is pick something that you can stick with longer than 2 weeks or a month.

Remember fad diets are just that a fad. Healthy weight management includes life style changes that last a lifetime. An example would be bread for me. I love bread with butter, brie cheese, bacon and cheese. However, I have chosen based upon my desire to have a healthy temple for God's service to have a BMI under 25 and to have bread on the weekends, not with every meal the way I used to and between meals, too.

One of the keys to health is flexibility, adapting and thriving through change and the dynamic brook of life.

If we follow the steps outlined in this book, prayer, studying God's Word, water, replacing the nutritional deficiencies, get moving, rest, relax, relate, release, moderation in eating and put our trust in God rather than people He will order our steps and let us focus on what He desires rather than just what we desire. What we will find is that our desires match His albeit at different times sometimes.

Reading this book is just the beginning, putting it into practice is the next step, allowing God to change your heart and mind through daily committing to spending time with HIM and hearing from HIM through HIS Word. You may not have a relationship with God and so you may say that it will not work, However, I challenge you to go into a room by yourself, ask God to forgive your sins, accept Him as Lord and Savior of your life and for the next 2 weeks teach you how to put the steps into practice.

Chapter 7

Putting it into practice for life— Final Thoughts Conclusion of the Whole Matter

Have you mastered it?…It takes at least 6 weeks of daily resolving to do it and consistently doing it so that you will see the benefits of your labor.

Follow the 10 steps. If you buy this book and you faithfully follow it, I don't mean with a twinkie in your mouth saying, Oh this book does not work because you want a side of doritos with onion dip on it or nachos dripping with cheese and extra meat sauce…if you faithfully follow the program for six weeks and you don't lose a pound and you don't have hypothyroidism, diabetes or another comorbid condition which prevents you from losing weight, you can personally call me and I will review your bariatric history and eating plan and discuss a program option for you.

The conclusion of the whole matter

This book is not a panacea. Obesity is a very complex elephant. This book represents one bite of the elephant because the studies are still being developed, the literature, and the knowledge related to all of the etiologic factors is still evolving.

It really comes down to a mindset change. The integration of the mind, body, and spirit. God gave us the wherewithal to fight this ongoing battle and win. The change agent cannot be external, it must be internal or the weight does not stay off. Healing has to occur from the inside out. It is not just about discipline. There are many people who are disciplined and still lose the same 25 pounds over and over again.

It is about praying and deciding to do it. Setting your heart on what really matters. First things first. Do this and your mind and body will follow. Eat to live and not live to eat as an anesthetic for today's problems. Today we live in a world of excess, affluence, have, or have not.

Either we are going to make an impact or we are not. Either we can run and jump with our children because we have the energy that God gave us or we are not. Either we love living or we don't. No more excuses. One step at a time, one foot in front of the other.

Just follow the steps consistently and see that it works. It is not a particular program because under the step of moderation in eating; they all work if you stick with them, It is about portion control, control of intake along with the other steps, not in lieu of the other steps, good health is the heart of the matter. It is not just about looking good on the outside, it about feeling good on the inside. The key is prayer because it releases the stress that so many of us carry because we cannot put it in place our selves and our way although we try. God can put situations and people together that you cannot imagine in ways that you cannot imagine if you are thankful and give Him the stress. Don't let stress do a slow boil. I was a stressed out overweight, overloaded doctor who did not represent health well. Sure I did not smoke and I expoused the rhetoric, however when people looked at me all they did not see a representative of health and wellness from the inside out. They saw excess in every way, weight, jewelry, makeup, excess to camouflage overwork and overload. This is my story and the practical tips that work.

Reading this book is just the beginning, putting it into practice is the next step, allowing God to change your heart and mind through daily committing to spending time with HIM and hearing from HIM through HIS Word. You may not have a relationship with God and so you may say that it will not work, However, I challenge you to go into a room by yourself, ask God to forgive your sins, accept Him as Lord and Savior of your life and for the next 2 weeks teach you how to put the steps into practice, I challenge you to email me at goodmedicinemd@yahoo.com and share your testimony.

It will work whether you are 5 pounds overweight or 100 pounds, I know, I was over 71 pounds overweight and went from 211 to 136.

Chapter 8

A new Beginning
Scriptures for Daily Practice

Daily Scripture List

Scriptures—Daily devotional and bedside prayer journal/thought list

1. Matthew 6:33—it's not about losing the weight, it's about what is weighing you down—Seek ye first the kingdom of God and his righteousness and all these things will be added unto you

2. Romans 8:28—Don't wig out, it will work out if you believe in Him

3. Proverbs17:22—Laughter is the best medi-cine A merry heart doeth good like a medi-cine, but a broken spirit drieth the bones. Cry

for a moment, pray to God, Believe in Faith get up wipe your tears and move forward

4. Set your heart to seek God in all you do including weight management 2 chronicles 11:16. Be consistent, write it down, and follow it and you will see results.

5. In all thy ways acknowledge him and he shall direct thy paths—ordered steps Proverbs 3, 5, 6,7, 8

6. Be anxious for nothing, prayer and supplication make your requests known to God—give your to do list to God. It cannot get all done in one day

7. Delight yourself in God and He will give you the desire of your heart

8. The peace of God; God shall keep your hearts and minds Philippians 4:7

9. A sound heart is the life of the flesh. Take care of your heart—Release envy and bitterness, they are the rottenness to the bones. It makes your heart sick

10. Keep thy heart with all diligence; for out of it are the issues of life, hurt, anger, bitterness, malice, unforgiveness which will weigh you

down and keep you out of balance. It is not about them forgiving, it is about you forgiving and not moving on, moving forward.

Remember to release control. All things work together for the good to them that love the Lord and are the called according to His purpose.

References/Supplemental Reading List

SOURCE: Wellness International Network Ltd—web.winltd.com

Life management for busy women

Holy Bible

CDC website—Division of Nutritional and Physical Activity

FDA website

The American Heritage Dictionary

978-0-595-39327-5
0-595-39327-6

www.ingramcontent.com/pod-product-compliance
Lightning Source LLC
Chambersburg PA
CBHW050336290526
45785CB00006B/2521